Patient with Acute Thoracic Myelopathy due to Degenerative Disease

Elements in Emergency Neurosurgery

DOI: 10.1017/9781009421553
First published online: May 2025

James M. W. Robins
Leeds General Infirmary

Deb Pal
Leeds General Infirmary

Author for correspondence: James M. W. Robins,
jmwrobins@doctors.org.uk

Abstract: Whilst thoracic myelopathy secondary to degenerative disease is relatively uncommon, left untreated it carries significant morbidity. It is thus of critical importance that patients are correctly diagnosed and managed expediently and effectively. Unfortunately, the management of thoracic myelopathy can be challenging, not least due to the technical difficulty accessing the site of compression, and indeed optimum management is also debated. In this Element the authors present background, clinical features, diagnosis, and pitfalls and then a handy management algorithm for this critical neurosurgical condition.

Keywords: thoracic myelopathy, thoracic disc, thoracic spinal stenosis, management, investigation

© James M. W. Robins and Deb Pal 2025

ISBNs: 9781009421546 (PB), 9781009421553 (OC)
ISSNs: 2755-0656 (online), 2755-0648 (print)

Contents

Introduction 1

Epidemiology, Background, and Aetiology
of Thoracic Myelopathy 1

Clinical Presentation of Thoracic Myelopathy 3

Principles of Diagnosis, Diagnostic Pitfalls,
and Role of Imaging 3

Management Strategies 5

Recommendations 6

References 7

Cambridge Elements

Elements in Emergency Neurosurgery
edited by
Nihal Gurusinghe
Lancashire Teaching Hospital NHS Trust
Peter Hutchinson
University of Cambridge, Society of British Neurological Surgeons and Royal College of Surgeons of England
Ioannis Fouyas
Royal College of Surgeons of Edinburgh
Naomi Slator
North Bristol NHS Trust
Ian Kamaly-Asl
Royal Manchester Children's Hospital
Peter Whitfield
University Hospitals Plymouth NHS Trust

PATIENT WITH ACUTE THORACIC MYELOPATHY DUE TO DEGENERATIVE DISEASE

James M. W. Robins
Leeds General Infirmary

Deb Pal
Leeds General Infirmary

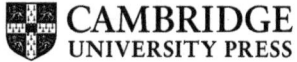

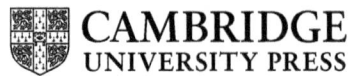

Shaftesbury Road, Cambridge CB2 8EA, United Kingdom

One Liberty Plaza, 20th Floor, New York, NY 10006, USA

477 Williamstown Road, Port Melbourne, VIC 3207, Australia

314–321, 3rd Floor, Plot 3, Splendor Forum, Jasola District Centre, New Delhi – 110025, India

103 Penang Road, #05–06/07, Visioncrest Commercial, Singapore 238467

Cambridge University Press is part of Cambridge University Press & Assessment, a department of the University of Cambridge.

We share the University's mission to contribute to society through the pursuit of education, learning and research at the highest international levels of excellence.

www.cambridge.org
Information on this title: www.cambridge.org/9781009421546

DOI: 10.1017/9781009421553

© James M. W. Robins and Deb Pal 2025

This publication is in copyright. Subject to statutory exception and to the provisions of relevant collective licensing agreements, no reproduction of any part may take place without the written permission of Cambridge University Press & Assessment.

When citing this work, please include a reference to the DOI 10.1017/9781009421553

First published 2025

A catalogue record for this publication is available from the British Library

ISBN 978-1-009-42154-6 Paperback
ISSN 2755-0656 (online)
ISSN 2755-0648 (print)

Cambridge University Press & Assessment has no responsibility for the persistence or accuracy of URLs for external or third-party internet websites referred to in this publication and does not guarantee that any content on such websites is, or will remain, accurate or appropriate.

For EU product safety concerns, contact us at Calle de José Abascal, 56, 1°, 28003 Madrid, Spain, or email eugpsr@cambridge.org

Every effort has been made in preparing this Element to provide accurate and up-to-date information which is in accord with accepted standards and practice at the time of publication. Although case histories are drawn from actual cases, every effort has been made to disguise the identities of the individuals involved. Nevertheless, the authors, editors and publishers can make no warranties that the information contained herein is totally free from error, not least because clinical standards are constantly changing through research and regulation. The authors, editors and publishers therefore disclaim all liability for direct or consequential damages resulting from the use of material contained in this Element. Readers are strongly advised to pay careful attention to information provided by the manufacturer of any drugs or equipment that they plan to use.

Introduction

Thoracic myelopathy secondary to degenerative disease is uncommon. However, if prompt diagnosis and management is not initiated, significant morbidity and functional deterioration results [1–4]. Following diagnosis, however, management can also be technically challenging. As such is it crucial that the neurosurgeon has an understanding of effective management for these patients. Here we present the clinical features, principles of diagnosis, and management options for this important neurosurgical condition (see Figure 1).

Epidemiology, Background, and Aetiology of Thoracic Myelopathy

Epidemiology

Estimation of incidence and prevalence of thoracic myelopathy is difficult as it is likely there is significant underdiagnosis [5]. Compression can be anterior due to thoracic disc herniation, with reported incidence of clinically significant disc herniation as 1 per 1 million people, representing 0.25% of all herniated discs [6, 7]. Posterior compression from ligamentum flavum thickening and facet joint hypertrophy are also important causes of myelopathy, representing 64% and 46% of causes in one study, respectively [8]. Surgical intervention, a surrogate of a likely highly conservative marker for the true prevalence of thoracic myelopathy, is reported as 0.9% per 100 000 in a Japanese study [9]. Of note is that this prevalence is less than 10% of the reported intervention for cervical myelopathy, and in reality, a true global incidence of prevalence is currently unclear [9, 10].

Background

The less-known incidence of thoracic myelopathy is likely due to underdiagnosis but also due to natural protection of the thoracic spine from degenerative changes. This is the result of limited movement in the thoracic spine due to the stabilising effect of the rib cage with consequently most degeneration occurring in the most mobile region below T8 [11, 12].

However, it is well appreciated that the thoracic spinal cord is highly sensitive to external insult. This is perhaps the result of relative poor vascularity especially at cranial and caudal vascular watershed areas and underlying individual cellular and genetic vulnerability [5, 13]. It thus follows that when the thoracic cord is subject to external compression, such as from degenerative disease, stenosis, or disc, or both, thoracic myelopathy ensues. As such, when thoracic myelopathy does occur, surgical intervention is usually required in a timely

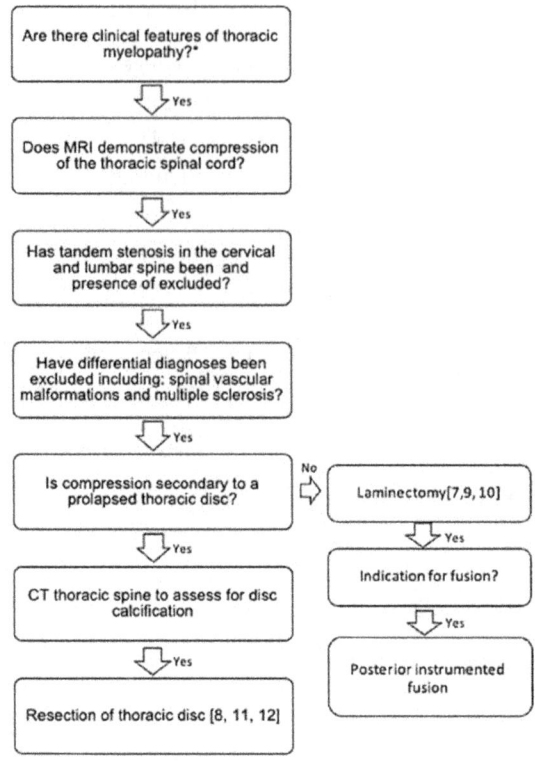

*Clinical features of thoracic myelopathy include[11, 15, 22, 36–40]:
Girdle pain
Back pain/low back pain
Leg numbness
Leg pain
Gait disturbance
Leg weakness
Spinal claudication
Bowel and bladder dysfunction
Hyperreflexia – patellar and ankle and upgoing plantar reflexes
Ankle clonus

Figure 1 Algorithm for the management of degenerative spinal cord compression.

manner, due to clinical progression and poor outcomes associated with conservative management [1–4].

Aetiology

The aetiology of degenerative thoracic myelopathy varies depending on populations. In Western populations, thoracic disc herniation is often reported as the commonest overall cause (95.7%), with ossified ligamentum flavum and ossified posterior longitudinal ligament (OPLL) less common at 3.6% and 0.5%%, respectively [13, 14]. The most common locations of disc herniations are caudal to T8 and at T11-12 [6, 15]. In Eastern populations, notably Japan, OPLL makes up a much larger cause (45%), with fewer thoracic disc herniations (2.1%) [16]. Interestingly, in the authors' experience, ligamental and facet hypertrophy are the most common causes of symptomatic thoracic myelopathy, particularly in patients over the age of 60 years, with thoracic discs representing a smaller proportion of cases [8].

Clinical Presentation of Thoracic Myelopathy

Diagnosis of thoracic myelopathy may be challenging, not least due to overlap of myelopathy or radiculopathy symptoms from cervical or lumbar spinal regions. Symptoms include lower limb and girdle pain, lower back pain, motor and sensory deficits, and bowel, bladder, and sexual dysfunction [11, 17]. Naturally, this overlap with other pathological spinal regions may delay diagnosis and thus increase morbidity [13, 18]. It is also of importance that thoracic cord pathology is occasionally confused with cardiac, pulmonary, or even abdominal pathology [19, 20].

Presentation may vary based on the site of compression. Radicular symptoms such as dermatomal chest wall discomfort or band-like pain result from posterolateral compression [10].

Central compression typically results in myelopathic features with long tract signs such as lower limb weakness, hypertonia, hyperreflexia, upgoing plantars, and clonus, with positive Rhomberg's sign and sometimes also sensory alteration. If severe, features of loss of bowel or bladder control with a sensory level in the trunk and incomplete/complete paraplegia may manifest [13, 17, 18].

Principles of Diagnosis, Diagnostic Pitfalls, and Role of Imaging

Sagittal and axial T2-weighted MRI is the initial imaging modality of choice for evaluation of spinal cord compression. It is also useful to perform MRI of the whole spine as this enables avoidance of missing cervical myelopathy, which can be a common pitfall (Figure 2) [13, 18, 21, 22]. MRI of whole spine also enables identification of the number of vertebrae, and appearance of any lumbarised or sacralised segments [21, 22]. This latter point is important if surgical treatment is subsequently indicated, to enable localisation of the correct operative level.

In cases of thoracic disc herniation, CT is necessary to assess the level of calcification as this pathology is often poorly appreciated on MRI (Figure 3) [21–24]. CT is also naturally useful in rare cases of OPLL-causing stenosis. For completeness, evaluation of sagittal balance in the form of standing lateral (and

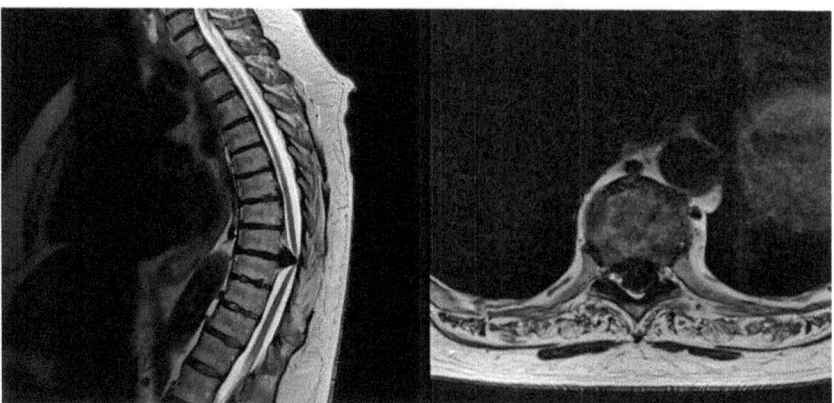

Figure 2 Sagittal and axial T2-weighted MRI demonstrating spinal cord compression from a large thoracic disc at the T8-9 level.

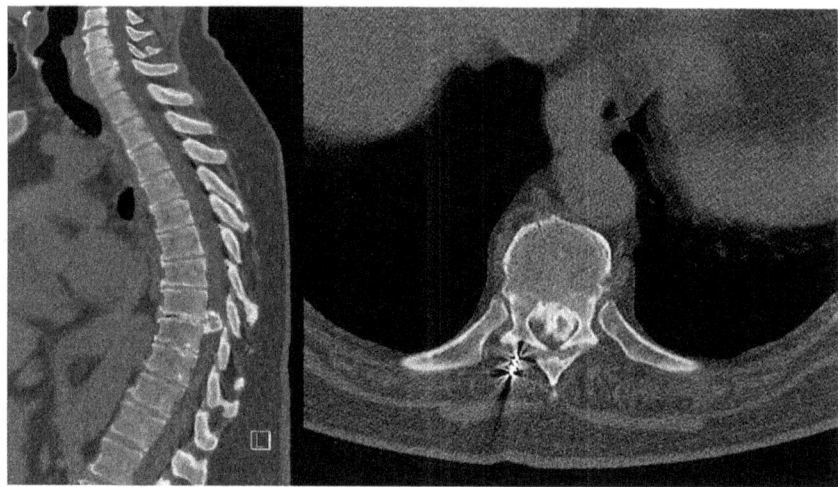

Figure 3 Sagittal and axial CT of the same patient imaged in Figure 1, demonstrating calcification of thoracic disc prolapse at T8-9. This emphasises the importance of pre-op CT evaluation as calcification is much better appreciated on CT than on MRI. Note also the presence of a pedicle marker on the axial image to aid swift intraoperative level localisation.

AP) X-ray of the thoracic spine is also useful prior to consideration of surgical fixation to prevent thoracic kyphosis progression [25].

The authors also advocate for the use of preoperative placement of CT-guided pedicle marker to avoid a common pitfall of operating at the incorrect level (Figure 3) [26]. This involves the placement of a radiopaque marker, such as an coil, in the pedicle of the intended operative level as guided by the CT. This enables quick, accurate localisation of the correct operative level and avoids time-consuming and increased radiation exposure of counting spinal levels using fluoroscopy from cervical or lumbar regions [27, 28].

Management Strategies

Management of thoracic canal stenosis from ligamental and bony thickening or OPLL is non-controversial as conservative management of symptomatic degenerative thoracic myelopathy is associated with poor neurological outcome. Hence, surgical management is frequently indicated [8, 10, 29]. Once cervical and lumbar pathologies have been excluded, surgical approach is based on the location of compression. Surgery necessitates a posterior decompression at the appropriate involved spinal level. Compared to the traditional laminectomy in the rest of the spine, laminectomy at the thoracic level can be more challenging given the increased sensitivity of the thoracic spinal cord with greater risk of neurological complications. If there is concern regarding instability due to interruption of the posterior tension band or need for a wider decompression with facetal removal, posterior instrumented fusion may be indicated.

However, the optimal management and approach for thoracic disc herniation is the subject of much debate with the description of several broad categories of approach, including anterior transthoracic, posterolateral, lateral extrapleural [30], and more recently the endoscopic approach [31, 32]. However, the antero lateral approach remains the gold standard.

Anterior approaches include traditional open thoracotomy or mini-variants and also thoracoscopic [30]. Posterolateral approaches include transfacetal, transpedicular, as well as minimally invasive tubular oblique paraspinal and endoscopic transforaminal approaches [30]. Lateral extrapleural approaches include tubular oblique retropleural and traditional open lateral extracavitatory approaches [30]. The authors' experience concur with the reported morbidity associated with traditional approaches, not least large incisions, rib resections, and blood loss [33–35].

As such we favour a minimally invasive direct lateral retropleural approach utilising mini-thoracotomy (approximately 5 cm). This combined with a tubular retractor system otherwise used in cases of lumbar extreme lateral interbody fusion XLIF® (NuVasive, San Diego, CA, USA) and the operative microscope enables effective access and visualisation to enable thoracic disc resection.

Due to the lack of evidence regarding optimum technique of thoracic disc resection, the authors recommend utilisation of techniques familiar to each institution. The authors also strongly advocate the use of intraoperative spinal monitoring.

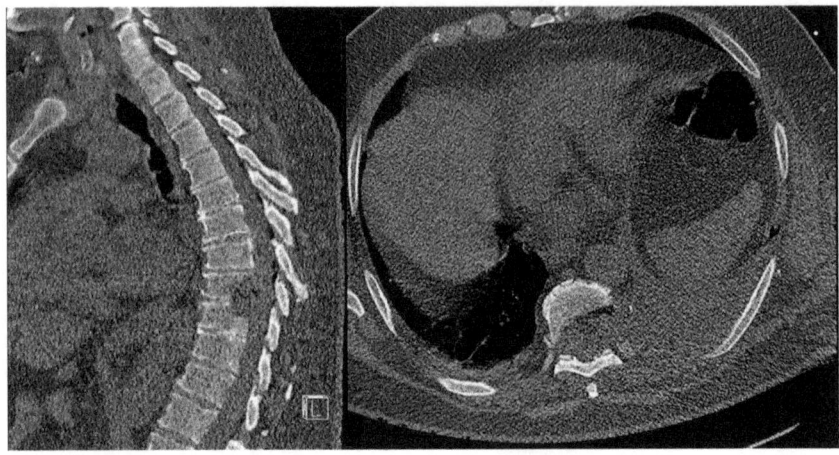

Figure 4 Post-operative sagittal and axial CT of the same patient in Figures 1 and 2 demonstrating resection of the thoracic disc prolapse with resection of the posterior aspects of T8 and T9 vertebral bodies. This procedure was performed via a minimally invasive direct lateral retropleural approach utilising mini-thoracotomy.

Recommendations

- The thoracic spinal cord is the least common region affected, but least resilient region to compression from degenerative disease thus resulting in thoracic myelopathy.
- Prompt diagnosis and exclusion of other sites of spinal cord compression, for example cervical, are crucial to enable prompt surgical management.
- Degenerative compression in Western populations is most likely due to thoracic disc prolapse and ligamental hypertrophy.
- Management of acute thoracic myelopathy secondary to degenerative disease is challenging.
- Thoracic discs are frequently calcified, thus preoperative CT evaluation is essential.

Management of thoracic disc prolapse is resection of the thoracic disc and management of ligamental thickening is laminectomy.

References

1. Kashyap S, Webb AG, Friis EA, Arnold PM (2021) Management of single-level thoracic disc herniation through a modified transfacet approach: A review of 86 patients. Surg Neurol Int 12: 338. https://doi.org/10.25259/SNI_94_2021.
2. Yoon WW, Koch J (2021) Herniated discs: When is surgery necessary? EFORT open Rev 6:526–530. https://doi.org/10.1302/2058-5241.6.210020.
3. Aizawa T, Sato T, Sasaki H, et al. (2007) Results of surgical treatment for thoracic myelopathy: Minimum 2-year follow-up study in 132 patients. J Neurosurg Spine 7:13–20. https://doi.org/10.3171/SPI-07/07/013.
4. Nakajima H, Watanabe S, Honjoh K, et al. (2021) Differences in clinical and radiological features of thoracic disc herniation presenting with acute progressive myelopathy. Eur Spine J 30:829–836. https://doi.org/10.1007/S00586-020-06485-6.
5. Davies BM, Mowforth O, Gharooni AA, et al. (2022) A new framework for investigating the biological basis of degenerative cervical myelopathy [AO Spine RECODE-DCM Research Priority Number 5]: Mechanical stress, vulnerability and time. Glob spine J 12:78S–96S. https://doi.org/10.1177/21925682211057546.
6. Greenberg M (2010) Handbook of Neurosurgery, 7th ed. Thieme, New York.
7. Deckey J (2003) Thoracic disc herniation. In Vincent J Devlin (ed.), Spine Secrets (p. 451). Hanley & Belfus, Philadelphia.
8. Chang UK, Choe WG, Chung CK, Kim HJ (2001) Surgical treatment for thoracic spinal stenosis. Spinal Cord 39:362–369. https://doi.org/10.1038/SJ.SC.3101174.
9. Aizawa T, Sato T, Tanaka Y, et al. (2006) Thoracic myelopathy in Japan: Epidemiological retrospective study in Miyagi Prefecture during 15 years. Tohoku J Exp Med 210:199–208. https://doi.org/10.1620/TJEM.210.199.
10. Rujeedawa T, Mowforth OD, Davies BM, et al. (2023) Degenerative thoracic myelopathy: A scoping review of epidemiology, genetics, and pathogenesis. Glob Spine J 14(5):1664–1677. https://doi.org/10.1177/21925682231224768/ASSET/IMAGES/LARGE/10.1177_2192568223124768-FIG3.JPEG.
11. Ando K, Imagama S, Kobayashi K, et al. (2019) Clinical features of thoracic myelopathy: A single-center study. JAAOS Glob Res Rev 3:e18.00090. https://doi.org/10.5435/JAAOSGLOBAL-D-18-00090.

12. Stillerman CB, Chen TC, Couldwell WT, et al. (1998) Experience in the surgical management of 82 symptomatic herniated thoracic discs and review of the literature. J Neurosurg 88:623–633. https://doi.org/10.3171/jns.1998.88.4.0623.
13. Rujeedawa T, Mowforth OD, Davies BM, et al. (2023) Degenerative thoracic myelopathy: A scoping review of epidemiology, genetics, and pathogenesis. Glob Spine J 14(5):1664–1677. https://doi.org/10.1177/21925682231224768.
14. Schulder M, Hirschfeld A (1988) Thoracic spinal canal stenosis. J Neurosurg 68:160–161. https://doi.org/10.3171/JNS.1988.68.1.0160.
15. Bouthors C, Benzakour A, Court C (2019) Surgical treatment of thoracic disc herniation: An overview. Int Orthop 43:807–816. https://doi.org/10.1007/S00264-018-4224-0.
16. Chen G, Fan T, Yang X, et al. (2020) The prevalence and clinical characteristics of thoracic spinal stenosis: A systematic review. Eur Spine J 29:2164–2172. https://doi.org/10.1007/S00586-020-06520-6.
17. Takenaka S, Kaito T, Hosono N, et al. (2014) Neurological manifestations of thoracic myelopathy. Arch Orthop Trauma Surg 134:903–912. https://doi.org/10.1007/S00402-014-2000-1.
18. Toribatake Y, Baba H, Kawahara N, et al. (1997) The epiconus syndrome presenting with radicular-type neurological features. Spinal Cord 35:163–170. https://doi.org/10.1038/SJ.SC.3100369.
19. Park JE, Chung ME, Song DH, Choi HS (2014) Inexplicable abdominal pain due to thoracic spinal cord tumor. Ann Rehabil Med 38:273–276. https://doi.org/10.5535/ARM.2014.38.2.273.
20. Hanna SS, Jewell R, Anker CJ, et al. (2022) Clinical reasoning: A 67-year-old woman with abdominal pain, constipation, and urinary retention. Neurology 99(3):117–122. https://doi.org/10.1212/WNL.0000000000200748.
21. Al-Mahfoudh R, Mitchell PS, Wilby M, et al. (2016) Management of giant calcified thoracic disks and description of the trench vertebrectomy technique. Glob Spine J 6:584–591. https://doi.org/10.1055/S-0035-1570087.
22. Court C, Mansour E, Bouthors C (2018) Thoracic disc herniation: Surgical treatment. Orthop Traumatol Surg Res 104:S31–S40. https://doi.org/10.1016/J.OTSR.2017.04.022.
23. Debnath UK, McConnell JR, Sengupta DK, et al. (2003) Results of hemivertebrectomy and fusion for symptomatic thoracic disc herniation. Eur Spine J 12:292–299. https://doi.org/10.1007/s00586-002-0468-9.
24. Schmidek HH, Sweet WH (2000) Surgical management of thoracic disc herniations. Schmidek & Sweet Operative Neurosurgical Techniques (pp. 2122–2131), 4th ed. New York: W.B. Saunders.

25. Morvan G, Mathieu P, Vuillemin V, et al. (2011) Standardized way for imaging of the sagittal spinal balance. Eur Spine J 20:602–608. https://doi.org/10.1007/S00586-011-1927-Y.
26. Hsiang J (2011) Wrong-level surgery: A unique problem in spine surgery. Surg Neurol Int 2:47. https://doi.org/10.4103/2152-7806.79769.
27. Binning MJ, Schmidt MH (2010) Percutaneous placement of radiopaque markers at the pedicle of interest for preoperative localization of thoracic spine level. Spine (Phila Pa 1976) 35:1821–1825. https://doi.org/10.1097/BRS.0B013E3181C90BDF.
28. Young RM, Prasad V, Wind JJ, et al. (2014) Novel technique for preoperative pedicle localization in spinal surgery with challenging anatomy. J Neurosurg Spine 20:400–403. https://doi.org/10.3171/2013.12.SPINE13477.
29. Matsuyama Y, Yoshihara H, Tsuji T, et al. (2005) Surgical outcome of ossification of the posterior longitudinal ligament (OPLL) of the thoracic spine: Implication of the type of ossification and surgical options. J Spinal Disord Tech 18:492–497. https://doi.org/10.1097/01.BSD.0000155033.63557.9C.
30. Sharma SB, Kim J-S (2019) A review of minimally invasive surgical yechniques for the management of thoracic disc herniations. Neurospine 16:24–33. https://doi.org/10.14245/ns.1938014.007.
31. Choi K, Eun S, Lee S, Lee H (2010) Percutaneous endoscopic thoracic discectomy; transforaminal approach. min – Minim Invasive Neurosurg 53:25–28. https://doi.org/10.1055/s-0029-1246159.
32. Wagner R, Telfeian AE, Iprenburg M, et al. (2016) Transforaminal endoscopic foraminoplasty and discectomy for the treatment of a thoracic disc herniation. World Neurosurg 90:194–198. https://doi.org/10.1016/j.wneu.2016.02.086.
33. Bartels RHMA, Peul WC (2007) Mini-thoracotomy or thoracoscopic treatment for medially located thoracic herniated disc? Spine (Phila Pa 1976) 32:E581–E584. https://doi.org/10.1097/BRS.0b013e31814b84e1.
34. Quint U, Bordon G, Preissl I, et al. (2012) Thoracoscopic treatment for single level symptomatic thoracic disc herniation: A prospective followed cohort study in a group of 167 consecutive cases. Eur Spine J 21:637–645. https://doi.org/10.1007/s00586-011-2103-0.
35. Strom RG, Mathur V, Givans H, et al. (2015) Technical modifications and decision-making to reduce morbidity in thoracic disc surgery: An institutional experience and treatment algorithm. Clin Neurol Neurosurg 133:75–82. https://doi.org/10.1016/j.clineuro.2015.03.014.
36. Chen Z-Q, Sun C-G (2015) Clinical guideline for treatment of symptomatic thoracic spinal stenosis. Orthop Surg 7(3):208–212. https://doi.org/10.1111/os.12190.

37. Kalfas IH (2000) Laminectomy for thoracic spinal canal stenosis. Neurosurg Focus 9:1–3. https://doi.org/10.3171/FOC.2000.9.4.3.
38. Siller S, Pannenbaecker L, Tonn JC, Zausinger S (2020) Surgery of degenerative thoracic spinal stenosis-long-term outcome with quality-of-life after posterior decompression via an uni- or bilateral approach. Acta Neurochir (Wien) 162:317–325. https://doi.org/10.1007/S00701-019-04191-X.
39. Cheng XK, Bian FC, Liu ZY, et al. (2020) A comparison study of percutaneous endoscopic decompression and posterior decompressive laminectomy in the treatment of thoracic spinal stenosis. BMC Musculoskelet Disord 21(1):717. https://doi.org/10.1186/S12891-020-03739-8.
40. Cornips EMJ, Janssen MLF, Beuls EAM (2011) Thoracic disc herniation and acute myelopathy: Clinical presentation, neuroimaging findings, surgical considerations, and outcome. J Neurosurg Spine 14:520–528. https://doi.org/10.3171/2010.12.SPINE10273.

Cambridge Elements ≡

Emergency Neurosurgery

Nihal Gurusinghe
Lancashire Teaching Hospital NHS Trust

Professor Nihal Gurusinghe is a Consultant Neurosurgeon at the Lancashire Teaching Hospitals NHS Trust. He is on the Executive Council of the Society of British Neurological Surgeons as the Lead for NICE (National Institute for Health and Care Excellence) guidelines relating to neurosurgical practice. He is also an examiner for the UK and International FRCS examinations in Neurosurgery.

Peter Hutchinson
University of Cambridge, Society of British Neurological Surgeons and Royal College of Surgeons of England

Peter Hutchinson BSc MBBS FFSEM FRCS(SN) PhD FMedSci is Professor of Neurosurgery and Head of the Division of Academic Neurosurgery at the University of Cambridge, and Honorary Consultant Neurosurgeon at Addenbrooke's Hospital. He is Director of Clinical Research at the Royal College of Surgeons of England and Meetings Secretary of the Society of British Neurological Surgeons.

Ioannis Fouyas
Royal College of Surgeons of Edinburgh

Ioannis Fouyas is a Consultant Neurosurgeon in Edinburgh. His clinical interests focus on the treatment of complex cerebrovascular and skull base pathologies. His academic endeavours concentrate in the field of cerebrovascular pathophysiology. His passion is technical surgical training, fulfilled in collaboration with the Royal College of Surgeons of Edinburgh. Finally, he pursues Undergraduate Neuroscience teaching, with a particular focus on functional Neuroanatomy.

Naomi Slator
North Bristol NHS Trust

Naomi Slator FRCS (SN) is a Consultant Spinal Neurosurgeon based at North Bristol NHS Trust. She has a specialist interest in Complex Spine alongside Cranial and Spinal Trauma. She completed her neurosurgical training in Birmingham and a six-month Fellowship in CSF and Trauma (2019). She then went on to complete her Spinal Fellowship in Leeds (2020) before moving to the southwest to take up her consultant post.

Ian Kamaly-Asl
Royal Manchester Children's Hospital

Ian Kamaly-Asl is a full time paediatric neurosurgeon and Honorary Chair at Royal Manchester Children's Hospital. He trained in North Western Deanery with fellowships at Boston Children's Hospital and Sick Kids in Toronto. Ian is a member of council of The Royal College of Surgeons of England and The SBNS where he is lead for mentoring and tackling oppressive behaviours.

Peter Whitfield
University Hospitals Plymouth NHS Trust

Professor Peter Whitfield is a Consultant Neurosurgeon at the South West Neurosurgical Centre, University Hospitals Plymouth NHS Trust. His clinical interests include vascular neurosurgery, neuro-oncology and trauma. He has held many roles in postgraduate neurosurgical education and is President of the Society of British Neurological Surgeons. Peter has published widely, and is passionate about education, training and the promotion of clinical research.

About the Series

Elements in Emergency Neurosurgery is intended for trainees and practitioners in Neurosurgery and Emergency Medicine as well as allied specialties all over the world. Authored by international experts, this series provides core knowledge, common clinical pathways and recommendations on the management of acute conditions of the brain and spine.

Cambridge Elements

Emergency Neurosurgery

Elements in the Series

Management of Seizures in Neurosurgical Practice
Julie Woodfield and Susan Duncan

Cranial and Spinal Tuberculosis Infections including Acute Presentations
Veekshith Shetty and Pragnesh Bhatt

Spinal Discitis and Epidural Abscess
Damjan Veljanoski and Pragnesh Bhatt

Adult Patient with Intraventricular, Paraventricular and Pineal Region Lesions
Mohamed Dablouk and Mahmoud Kamel

Ruptured Supratentorial Cerebral Artery Aneurysm with Large Intracerebral Haematoma
Samuel Hall and Diederik Bulters

Neurosurgical Handovers and Standards for Emergency Care
Simon Lammy and Jennifer Brown

Spontaneous Intracranial Haemorrhage Caused by a Non-aneurysmal Brain Vascular Malformation
Sherif R. W. Kirollos and Ramez W. Kirollos

Emergency Scenarios in Functional Neurosurgery
James Manfield and Nicholas Park

Management of a Patient with a Venous Sinus Thrombosis with or without an Intracerebral Haematoma
Helen Sims and James Choulerton

Patient with Suspected Cauda Equina Syndrome
Gabriel Metcalf-Cuenca and Patrick F. X. Statham

Assessment of a Patient in Coma
Alexander Shah and Holly Roy

Patient with Acute Thoracic Myelopathy due to Degenerative Disease
James M. W. Robins and Deb Pal

A full series listing is available at: www.cambridge.org/EEMN

For EU product safety concerns, contact us at Calle de José Abascal, 56–1°,
28003 Madrid, Spain or eugpsr@cambridge.org.

www.ingramcontent.com/pod-product-compliance
Lightning Source LLC
Chambersburg PA
CBHW071436090725
29362CB00008B/39